Botox: The Truth About Botox Injections

I0421561

An Introductory Guide to Botulinum Toxin Procedures, Costs, Options, and What You Must Know

Table of Contents

Introduction

In modern-day society, many consider looking young and beautiful a personal responsibility, along with getting a regular haircut or dressing in a presentable way. For better or worse, people seem to be more conscious of their appearance now than ever before.

Because the pressure to look good is at an all-time high, many have turned to cosmetic procedures to supplement their natural beauty and to attempt to halt the ever-ticking clock of aging. Botulinum toxin injections, more commonly known as Botox injections, are among these cosmetic procedures. In the following pages of this short and concise book, we will take a look at information on this topic.

This short book discusses what Botox actually *is*, as well as the cost of treatment, the history of the drug, its advantages and disadvantages, and more. We'll even go beyond cosmetics and delve into the medicinal uses of Botox, and a list of medical conditions that can be treated by this drug is presented in later chapters.

By the end of this book, you will have the necessary information to decide whether or not it is worth it to get Botox injections, for whatever your reasons. The content here isn't meant to be a form of medical advice, as this book is meant for informational purposes only. In this book we are aiming to look at this topic in an unbiased light. We are not promoting the use of Botox injections, per se, but we want to make sure that if someone is interested in this controversial topic, he or she can reach more informed conclusions.

We hope that you are able to learn a thing or two from   reading   this!

Chapter 1:

What Is Botox and How Much Is It?

One of the most widely known cosmetic treatments in the world is **Botox**. In 2012 alone, an estimated 6.2 million people underwent cosmetic procedures involving Botox, and the numbers are expected to have risen since then. But what *is* Botox, really? What does it do? Is it only for cosmetic purposes? Let's clear this up.

Defining Botox

Botox is actually a commercial brand name of a drug. It is administered through injection. It contains a substance called **botulinum toxin**, which is made from a neurotoxin produced by bacteria, called *Clostridium botulinum*. A few other species from the *Clostridium* family also produce this toxin. These bacteria can cause a frequently fatal type of food poisoning called botulism.

In its raw form, botulinum toxin can be dangerous—it is the most severely lethal toxin known to man. According to scientists' estimates, one gram could be enough to kill one million people, and several kilos would suffice to drive the human race to extinction.

But even with this potential for danger, why is there such a high demand for Botox? The answer is simple: it's effective.

"The dose makes the poison," or so the old adage goes, and this is true for botulinum toxin. When administered in the right dosage, with the right method, it is beneficial in a variety of ways.

In addition to a very, *very*, small dosage, commercial botulinum toxin has also been "purified" by pharmaceutical companies. They are approved by the FDA and do not have life-threatening side effects when administered correctly.

Approved Therapeutic Uses

Although it is now popular as a cosmetic treatment to lessen lines and wrinkles, botulinum toxin has actually been used as a treatment for **neurologic and ophthalmologic disorders** for over 20 years. It has been shown to be both relatively safe and effective.

The FDA has approved Botox to cure migraines, involuntary muscle spasms of the eyes and limbs, urinary incontinence, and excessive sweating. Aside from curing these conditions, Botox also has a number of off-label uses. However, these have not been evaluated and approved by the FDA. They may pose unanticipated risks to health and safety.

How Much Does It Cost?

Botox injections are less expensive than most cosmetic and medical procedures. However, Botox is not permanent. The effects typically last for 3 to 4 months, very rarely reaching 6 months. To continue reaping the benefits, one must pay for regular treatments indefinitely, so it can still be quite costly in the long run.

For Cosmetic Purposes

According to data from the American Society of Plastic Surgeons, the average cost of cosmetic procedures involving botulinum injections is **around $380**. This is not inclusive of miscellaneous expenses.

This average is typically the total of (1) the cost of the prescription, (2) payment for the surgeon or the person who administers the drug, and (3) the expenses of the facility treatment where it is administered. However, this is just an average. The costs of procedures vary greatly depending on a number of factors. There are two ways that offices compute the charge for Botox injections: by **area** or by **unit**.

In the by area approach, a client pays a set amount for a specific area. For example, a clinic may charge $250 for the forehead and $300 for frown lines. Offices that hold sales and discount specials on Botox frequently use this approach. They may charge as little as $150 per area, for example.

In the by unit approach, a client pays for the amount of Botox actually used. This amount is measured in units. The price for each unit may differ from place to place, but typically ranges from $10-15.

The number of units used also varies, as it depends on the facial area and severity of the lines. For one area, the amount of Botox used can be anywhere from 5 to 30 units.

Although the by area approach may seem more economical, many professionals actually advise against it. The main reason is because with this approach there is no way to know how much Botox has actually been used relative to the price.

For example, a rate of $150 per area may seem like a great discount, but if the shop with this offer uses 10 units or less for the procedure, then it amounts to $15/unit or more, which is not such a great deal after all. Also, with fewer units, the effect is less pronounced and will wear off sooner.

To get more value out of a budget, it is best to go with a facility with a by unit approach, or to make it a point to ask how many units of Botox will be used when opting for the alternative.

For Medical Purposes

The cost of Botox injections for medical purposes (like alleviating migraines and involuntary spasms) can be significantly higher than those of cosmetic treatments. This is because a considerably larger dosage is required. As previously mentioned, cosmetic procedures only use around 5-30 units. While dosage varies for medical treatments, it is usually significantly greater than this amount—often going over 100 units. Botox injections for medical purposes are typically priced per unit.

Botulinum Toxin Types and Brand Names

Botox is not the only drug to contain botulinum toxin, but it was the first. These days, there are newer products on the market. Be warned, though, as these brands are not identical and cannot be substituted for each other. The units used to measure them are not the same. They may also differ in the type of botulinum toxin they contain.

There are 7 different types of botulinum toxin. Of these different types, only type A and B are marketed as medical drugs. The FDA has emphasized the difference between brands by giving them different generic names. The types have also been indicated. Rest assured that they are all relatively safe when used in the proper manner.

Here are the brand names of drugs containing botulinum toxin and their respective generic names:

Botox, **Botox Cosmetic**, and **Vistabel**also known as OnabotulinumtoxinA, classified as botulinum toxin type A

Dysport also known as AbobotulinumtoxinA, classified as botulinum toxin type A

Xeomin and **Bocouture** also known as IncobotulinumtoxinA, classified as botulinum toxin type A

Myobloc also known as RimabotulinumtoxinB, classified botulinum toxin type B

Finally, remember that all these drugs are licensed as **prescription medication**. They should **only** be used when approved by a physician and administered by a medical professional.

Chapter 2:

A History of Botulinum Toxin and Botox

These days, Botox and its competitors are household names, more or less. Also, just like with many modern day conveniences, it is rare for people to think about their origin or even to wonder how they came to be.

Like many medical discoveries, botulinum toxin has had a rich and fascinating history. *How exactly did a lethal poison become one of the most commonly used drugs around the world?* Let's go over a brief account of the discovery and development of botulinum toxin over the decades.

In the 1800's: It All Started with Sausage

The year is 1820 and Dr. Justinus Kerner is studying blood sausages. Seems strange, doesn't it? But these weren't your average sausages— these had caused the death of a couple dozen Germans. Kerner was convinced that something inside these spoiled sausages caused disease and subsequent death.

His studies led to the discovery of botulinum toxin, a detailed analysis of its effects on the human body, and a more comprehensive knowledge of food poisoning in general. He was also the first to consider botulinum toxin for therapeutic use.

Seven decades later, Belgian scientist Dr. Emile van Ermengem discovered that the toxin was produced by a certain species of bacteria, and this pathogen is now known as *Clostridium botulinum*.

From the 1940's to the 1960's: Bioweapons and Benefits

As previously mentioned, botulinum toxin is among the most dangerous substances in the world. It should come as no surprise that efforts were made to study its potential as a biological weapon. This began in the 1940's with the onset of World War II.

Some of the warring countries came up with plans to assassinate enemies with the toxin. One such plan involved Chinese prostitutes slipping botulinum toxin pills into the food and drink of high-profile Japanese officers. The pills were actually produced, but the plan was never executed.

After the war, research shifted from how botulinum toxin could kill people to how it could help them. Dr. Vernon Brooks, a physiologist, first discovered the "relaxing" effect of botulinum toxin type A on hyperactive muscles in 1953.

Taking note of this effect, ophthalmologist Dr. Alan B. Scott thought it could be used to treat strabismus (crossed eyes). Scott began testing the drug on monkeys in the 60's.

From the 70's and 80's: "Botox" is Born

The FDA finally gave Dr. Scott approval for human testing in 1978. Botulinum toxin was injected into volunteers with strabismus. By the 1980's, Scott had published numerous studies on the results. He came to the conclusion that the toxin was a successful and safe treatment for strabismus.

Subsequent research uncovered even more possible uses for botulinum toxin, especially against involuntary muscle contractions of numerous kinds: facial spasms to spasms of the vocal cord.

In 1988, the pharmaceutical company, Allergan, acquired the rights to distribute Scott's batch of botulinum toxin type A, then known as "Oculinum." The next year, the FDA officially sanctioned the use of the toxin to treat strabismus and blepharospasms (eyelid spasms). After this, Allergan changed the drug's name from "Oculinum" to the now ubiquitous "Botox."

The 90's: Botox Becomes an Off-Label Miracle

The discovery of Botox as a cosmetic treatment was actually completely accidental.

Dr. Jean Carruthers was a Canadian ophthalmologist who was using Botox injections to treat patients with blepharospasm. Over time, she noticed that their frown lines were gradually softening and becoming less pronounced.

Building on this startling observation, she coordinated with her husband (who was a dermatologist) and published a study together in 1992. They concluded that although the effects were temporary, injecting Botox was a safe and easy method for treating brow wrinkles.

The FDA had not approved this use of Botox, but many dermatologists began to take advantage of this "off-label" purpose of the drug. By 1997, so many people were using Botox that supplies ran out all over the United States. There was a brief panic among its patrons until a new batch was produced and approved.

2000 and Onward: New Millennium, New Approvals

It would seem that the FDA took the dawn of the new millennium as a go-ahead for approving even more usages of Botox. They officially declared the drug as a treatment for cervical dystonia (spasms of the shoulder and neck) in 2000, followed by the long-awaited approval of it as a wrinkle-remover in 2002. In 2004, Botox was also accepted as an official treatment for axillary hyperhidrosis (excessive sweating of the underarms). It became a valid option for treating chronic migraines in 2010 and was presented as a cure for urinary incontinence and bladder problems in 2011.

Currently, there are many other "off-label" uses for Botox. However, is not unlikely that these will be approved in the future.

Chapter 3:

The Effects of Botox and The Science Behind It

The previous chapters have somewhat skimmed the surface of what botulinum toxin and Botox can do. Now let's get into the science behind it.

Treatments with the drug are generally successful, but there *are* side effects. Most of these are mild, but although it is extremely unlikely, there is a possibility for life-threatening complications to arise.

FDA Approved Cosmetic and Medical Uses

Currently, the FDA sanctions the use of drugs with botulinum toxin, including Botox, in treating a number of conditions listed below. Some of these have already been touched upon in the previous chapters.

Bear in mind that effects are **temporary** in all cases and will wear off after an average of 3 to 4 months.

For Cosmetic Use Against:

Glabellar lines, frown lines found between eyebrows. Treatment is for adults under 65 years of age.

Canthal lines, commonly called "crow's feet."

An increasing number of young adults in their 20's are getting Botox as a preventive measure. They believe this will help prevent wrinkles from appearing in the future.

Although there is no official age requirement for getting cosmetic Botox injections (other than being below 65), many experts agree that these twentysomethings don't need it, and they disapprove of Botox as a preventive measure.

Most plastic surgeons and dermatologists only advise Botox to their patients when wrinkles and lines are visible while the face it at rest, i.e. not grimacing or smiling. These patients are usually in their 40's and 50's.

For Medical Use Against:

Blepharospasm: involuntary twitching or spasms of the eyelids. Treatment is limited to those who are 12 years old and older.

Strabismus: misalignment of the eyes (commonly called "crossed eyes"). Treatment is only for individuals 12 years old and older.

Cervical dystonia: a neuromuscular disorder characterized by severe spasms of the neck and shoulder muscles. It causes someone's head to jolt to one side uncontrollably. Treatment is for individuals 16 years old and older.

Upper limb spasticity: involuntary muscle contractions of the upper limbs. It causes stiffness in finger, wrist, and elbow muscles. Treatment is for adults 18 years old and older.

Chronic migraine: characterized by the frequency and duration of migraines and a patient's history. Generally, a person experiences headaches for more than 15 days a month, each lasting 4 hours or more. Treatment is for adults 18 years old and older.

Overactive bladder: problems with the bladder's storage function. It causes sudden, frequent, and incontrollable urges to urinate, leading to incontinence. Treatment is for adults 18 years and older, and only when prior medication has had no effect.

Detrusor over activity leading to urinary incontinence: a neurologic condition involving the involuntary contraction of the bladder muscle. This leads to incontinence. Treatment is for adults 18 years and older, and it is only allowed when prior medication has had no effect or when side effects are intolerable.

Severe primary axillary hyperhidrosis: excessive sweating of the underarms due to unknown causes. Treatment is allowed only when topical medicines have not worked, and only for adults 18 years old and older.

For all these purposes, brands containing botulinum toxin type A (refer to Chapter 1), such as Botox, Botox Cosmetic, Vistabel, Dysport, Xeomin and Bocouture, can be used. The FDA has expressly indicated that botulinum toxin type B, marketed under the brand Myobloc, should only be used to treat cervical dystonia.

The Science Behind Botox

To understand the scientific mechanisms that allow Botox and similar drugs to work, one needs to understand the relationship between muscles and nerves.

A muscle contracts when a nerve sends it a signal to do so. The signal travels to the end of the nerve and reaches a gap between the nerve and the muscle, referred to as the **neuromuscular junction**. Once the signal reaches that point, a chemical named **acetylcholine** is released from the end of the nerve and binds to receptors on the muscle. This starts a series of reactions that causes the muscle to contract.

Drugs with botulinum toxin block the muscles' acetylcholine receptors. When the muscle cannot detect acetylcholine, no contraction occurs. Basically, the muscle becomes paralyzed because it cannot receive the signal for movement, even though there is no damage to it or to the nerves. This blockage of acetylcholine cannot be reversed and will begin 48 hours upon injection of the drug.

Why Does It Help?

Muscle paralysis may not seem like a good thing at first glance, but for those who suffer from *too much* muscle contraction, it may be the only way to relax overactive muscles and stop uncontrollable movement.

The paralysis of specific muscles helps stop the twitching and spasms caused by many diseases. It relaxes tense muscles that contribute to migraines and stops incontinence by preventing bladder muscles from contracting. The same principle applies to wrinkles and lines, as they become more obvious when muscles contract, so relaxing these muscles prevents wrinkles from being visible. Other wrinkles are results of permanent creasing on the skin. These cannot be erased totally, but they can be softened by treatment.

Why Is It Temporary?

Although the blocked acetylcholine receptors can never be "unblocked," new ones can develop in their place. Once new receptors develop, acetylcholine will be detected again and muscle contraction will resume. This process is usually completed at around 3 to 5 months. When enough new receptors are present, the effects of the medication will wear off, and involuntary muscle spasms will start again and wrinkles will begin   to   show.

Side Effects and Complications

Although the FDA *has* approved it, botulinum toxin is still a dangerous chemical. Mild side effects are unavoidable and even the sellers of Botox and other brands acknowledge this fact.

The safety information included in every package of Botox is very forthcoming. The benefits and dangers associated with the medication are also made very clear. According to this information, possible side effects include:

Difficulty breathing, speaking, or swallowing

This is due to the weakening of the muscles. The risk is higher if problems already exist prior to treatment. Symptoms can last for as long as several months, and they can also be severe and result in death.

Allergic reactions

A few patients have had allergic reactions to the drug, ranging from mild to severe. Symptoms include reactions on the skin, such as redness, itching, the appearance of welts and rashes. Asthma symptoms, wheezing, dizziness and feeling faint have also been reported. Also, symptoms can be immediate. If symptoms arise, then use of the drug should be stopped.

Cornea problems

Some patients receiving treatment for blepharospasm have reported problems of the cornea. Certain nerve disorders seem to increase the risk of this occurring. A possible reason is that the medication causes a person to blink less, thereby exposing the eye to more air than usual.

Bleeding in the back of the eye

Some patients being treated for strabismus have reported bleeding behind their eyeballs.

Common colds and bronchitis

Patients treated with Botox injections for upper limb spasticity have more frequent reports of bronchitis and common colds. The risk is greater for those who already have breathing-related issues prior to treatment.

Autonomic dysreflexia

This is a clinical syndrome that results in the sudden onset of dangerously high blood pressure. It is potentially fatal and is regarded as a medical emergency. This condition has been observed in patients treated with Botox for overactive bladders due to neurological causes.

Limits the range of facial expressions

This is obviously a side effect of cosmetic use. To remove lines and wrinkles, the facial muscles are effectively paralyzed. The lines and wrinkles are softened and the face has a more youthful look. However, this may come at the expense of one's facial expressions. Because the muscles are paralyzed, they cannot move to make expressions as clearly as before. Usually it is still possible to convey emotion despite these limitations, although there are extreme cases where the result is a "robotic" look due to excessive muscle paralysis.

Other side effects include: pain or discomfort at the site of injection, headache, dry mouth, neck pain, and tiredness. Eye problems such as blurred vision, double vision, dry eyes, decreased eyesight, swelling of eyelids and drooping eyelids have also been documented. Bladder problems such as painful urination, urinary tract infection, and the inability to empty the bladder have been documented.

Of course, not everyone experiences side effects, and this list simply presents the possibilities. The average person experiences only a fraction of these symptoms. In fact, many people who get Botox injections for cosmetic purposes only experience mild discomfort at most. They get the treatment and then continue on with their day as if nothing had happened. People who get injections for medical purposes may experience more pronounced side effects because they've received a higher dosage of botulinum toxin.

However, the final verdict is that the reactions are different for each person. There is no way to predict what side effects will be experienced until a person actually decides to have the treatment.

Complications and How to Avoid Them

Aside from the minor side effects, there is also a possibility of life-threatening complications. From 1989 to 2003, the FDA has identified 28 deaths due to complications caused by Botox and other brands of botulinum toxin. Although none of these deaths were due to cosmetic use, the risk still remains.

A major concern is that the effects of the toxin will spread to other areas of the body (not just the part that was injected). The possibility of this happening is small, but it is still a possibility, nonetheless. In the event that this does occur, the symptoms can be varied. These include, but are not limited to, difficulty breathing, trouble swallowing, an overall feeling of weakness and loss of strength, incontrollable drooping of eyelids, blurred vision or double vision, loss or hoarseness of voice, problems with articulation and speaking, and loss of bladder control.

Respiratory failure may be severe enough to result in death.

Fortunately, there have been no confirmed cases where the spread of the toxin was severe enough to be fatal. To further ensure safety and avoid complications, those intending to get botulinum toxin injections should respect the following guidelines:

Do not use the drug if you are allergic to any of its components.

Examine the ingredients before consenting to treatment. If an allergic reaction has been observed in the use of one brand, then do not try a different brand. The allergic reaction will probably occur again.

Inform a doctor of existing nerve or muscle conditions prior to treatment.

Conditions like Lou Gehrig's disease or ALS, Lambert-Eaton syndrome, and myasthenia gravis may increase the risk of serious side effects.

Inform a doctor of breathing-related issues prior to treatment.

This is especially significant for those with upper limb spasticity and detrusor over activity because the risk of unwanted pulmonary effects have been shown to increase when people with these conditions undergo treatment.

Inform a doctor of all medical conditions prior to treatment.

This will help the doctor evaluate the overall safety of the procedure for a patient. All medical issues before treatment should be known, as well as any future medical treatments and procedures planned, such as surgery.

Inform a doctor of all medication taken prior to and during the treatment.

This should include all drugs ingested, whether they are prescription, nonprescription, vitamins, or herbal supplements. Certain medicines can increase the risk of major side effects when paired with botulinum toxin. Also, do not start any type of medication after treatment without consulting a doctor first. This guideline is especially important when antibiotic injections, sleeping medicine, muscle relaxants, anti-coagulants or anti-platelets (like aspirin), and cold or allergy medicine is involved.

Inform a doctor of any other botulinum toxin products used in the past.

A doctor should know if a patient has had prior experience with botulinum toxin. The purpose and brand of the medication should be indicated. Any injections of the drug in the last four months should be reported prior to treatment.

Do not use the drug if you are pregnant or planning a pregnancy.

Do not use the drug if you are breastfeeding or planning to breastfeed.

By following the correct dosage and adhering to guidelines and the appropriate procedures, it is possible to reap the benefits of these medications with only minimum side effects. Remember to always get treatments from reputable medical professionals who can ensure the success and safety of these procedures.

Do not be blinded by cheaper prices or easier methods of purchase—via the Internet, for example. Always have your cosmetic or medical procedures performed by well-informed and licensed professionals.

Chapter 4:

The Pros and Cons of Botox Injections

The previous chapters have outlined the positive and negative effects of Botox and other drugs containing botulinum toxin. It is now up to the person who will undergo the procedure to weigh the advantages against the risks and decide for or against getting injections.

The information presented earlier on may have been a bit overwhelming. To help you take stock of what has been discussed so far, this chapter clearly illustrates the pros and cons of getting botulinum toxin injections.

The Pros

1. It is effective.

There's no denying the effectiveness of these treatments. Whether it is for cosmetic or medical use, when the treatment is performed properly the results are almost always guaranteed to be satisfying.

For those who use it cosmetically and for aesthetic purposes, the confidence gained is significant indeed. It allows people to have a sort of self-assurance that will undoubtedly affect their overall happiness and state of mind. For those who use it for medical purposes, the relief must be immense. To be freed from distracting and embarrassing medical symptoms does wonders in improving the comfort and overall quality of life of these patients.

2. It is relatively affordable in the short term.

Compared to other cosmetic and medical procedures, botulinum toxin injections certainly cost less per treatment. All things considered, $10-15/unit is a reasonable price to pay for the potential benefits, especially if your looks are crucial to your career. Many offices and clinics even have discounts or sales that bring the price down even further. More importantly, no price can pay for the comfort, confidence, and improved sense of self that these injections can give to some people - whatever purpose they may be using it for.

3. It is easy and non-invasive.

Just one injection and it's done! The procedure itself takes no more than an hour at a time and a long and drawn-out recovery time is not necessary. It doesn't require extensive preparation, whether from the one getting the treatment or the one administering it. This saves time, resources, and money.

For a quick and easy fix of the conditions it can treat, one would be hard-pressed to find something better than botulinum toxin injections.

4. It is easy to find.

Lastly, because it is so popular, there is no shortage in providers of the treatment. Patients can have their pick of facilities while keeping in mind the price and skill of personnel, among other considerations. The competition also results to better prices for the people getting the treatment, as many practices lower their prices in an attempt to attract more customers and outmatch their competitors.

Competition is healthy for businesses *and* customers in a lot of ways. Just remember to not be swayed too quickly by low prices. Paying a little extra for better quality is always preferable to paying cheap and then spending more trying to fix a "botched" job. As with many other commercial goods, the maxim, "you get what you pay for," applies.

The Cons

1. It is temporary.

As previously explained, botulinum toxin injections are temporary and the effects usually last an average of 3 to 4 months. The duration varies from person to person, but there's no escaping the fact that to maintain the effect, subsequent treatments are a necessity. This leads to the second disadvantage on this list.

2. It costs a lot in the long term.

Although these treatments are relatively inexpensive, the fact that one has to keep maintaining them will inevitably lead to more expenses. The costs can add up over the years and may eventually prove to be too much to continue indefinitely.

Of course, one could always stop treatment, but the truth is no one wants to be treated for something only to have it come back. No one wants to be wrinkle-free for a time only to go back to having wrinkles once that period is over.

3. It can have many side effects

These side effects have all been outlined in Chapter 3. They are an inevitable part of the treatment and may affect some people more than others. Although there are steps to reduce the risks of these side effects, there is no way to guarantee that they will not occur. The potential for danger may be low, but it *is* there. People should have that fact in mind as they consent to these treatments.

4. It has many practitioners.

This is basically the flipside of the fourth advantage listed in the "Pros" section. Although more practitioners mean better availability, it cannot be denied that some of these *"practitioners"* are actually not very skilled or even qualified for the job.

Because sub-par practitioners usually charge lower-than-average rates, they still manage to attract a great number of customers. Sadly, a lot of these customers end up dissatisfied with the results or, worse, get botched jobs that lower their confidence instead of raising it.

To avoid falling victim to these cons, research and investigate thoroughly before deciding to who and where to have treatments done.

Conclusion

Thank you for reading this! We hope this short, concise book was able to teach you a thing or two about the intriguing topic of Botox injections.

Now that you understand the important factors regarding Botox, you can decide if you want to try it, or if you can inform your friends who ask you about it. Plus, a little addition to your knowledge doesn't hurt, right? Our world is becoming increasingly interested in the use of aesthetic aides, whether it be for sex changes, physical transformations, or just a little touch up help.

If you've learned anything from this book, please take the time to share your thoughts by sending me a message or even posting a review to Amazon.

Thank you and good luck in your journey!